The One Exercise Solution: *Maximum Results with Minimum Effort*

Bill Gallagher PT, CMT, CYT

Bill Gallagher PT, CMT, CYT

ISBN:
ISBN-13:

DEDICATION

**To my patients & colleagues who I have learned so much from.
Jessica, Jaya & Melia for their love and support.**

Table of Contents

Chapter 1: Introduction

Exercise is the closest thing to a "fountain of youth" that we know of so far. Almost every day a new scientific study is published indicating the benefits of exercise that include:

1. Improving or maintaining functional ability.
2. Improving balance.
3. Preventing falls.
4. Improving mood, decreasing depression.
5. Improving body composition (less fat, more muscle, and denser bone).
6. Improving ability to deal with physical and mental stress.
7. Improving sleep quality (which in turn improves mood, cognition, eating habits, immune function).
8. Improving cognition and preventing or delaying the onset of dementia.
9. Improving sexual function.

As a physical therapist, I put a huge value on the first item on the list above: Maintaining or improving function for myself and my patients. Exercise that works muscles and burns calories, but does **not** improve or maintain functional ability is WAY less interesting and important than exercise that is functionally meaningful. Unfortunately, many exercises that I see recommended for elders are totally non-functional. One of the most important abilities to maintain or develop is standing up from a chair, toilet or bed. Over the course of my career working with patients in the hospital right after surgery or illness and when they get home, I have worked with scores if not hundreds of people who were not able to toilet themselves without help. Very often these people needed help not to walk or wipe themselves, but needed help STANDING UP FROM A CHAIR.
Unless I am crushed by a giant asteroid or run over by a truck, there will likely come a day when I am unable to toilet myself. Given my experience, I know that is most likely to be because I am unable to stand up from a chair, bed or toilet seat (usually the lowest seat in the home). I would like to "kick" that day "as far down the street" into the future as possible. I bet you would like to do that too. Developing surplus strength, flexibility and skill in sit↔stand is a surefire way to keep that day from coming prematurely.

Who is this book for?

1. People who have very limited time to exercise.
2. People who have trouble staying motivated to exercise.
3. People who have trouble exercising safely on their own due to balance issue or other limitations.
4. People who are having trouble getting up and down from a chair, couch, car seat or toilet.
5. People who are losing strength and balance and want to stop and reverse this loss.
6. Family members of non-exercisers hoping to influence their loved one to do something to slow down or stop functional decline.
7. Physicians, Physical Therapists, Occupational Therapists and fitness professionals looking to improve their ability to get their patients to do a key functionally relevant exercise.

This book will help you to use this one exercise to build strength in the whole body, improve your muscular and cardiovascular endurance, flexibility in key joints & muscle groups and get all the benefits of exercise listed above. I will guide you on improving your "form" and finding ease, comfort and even pleasure in this exercise. I will map out when to do it, how often, how to progress yourself and when to give it a rest. I will show you tricks to make standing up easier if you are having trouble getting up. I will also show you how to make it harder and vary the challenge to keep you progressing when it gets easy. The chapter on the pelvis and how to move it for maximum efficiency will help improve posture, build core strength and awareness and decrease pain while further improving your ability to do the exercise smoothly and efficiently. The chapter on breathing will help you use the breathing muscles to work with you (rather than against you) when you are doing the exercise. Finally, Chapter 9: Where is the Mind, will turn this exercise into a meditation in movement giving you all the benefits that a meditation practice has been shown to deliver. Along with clear explanations of all the above, you will have photos to illustrate all the information, access to handouts and a log that you can print out and use to remind yourself (or your loved one, patient or client) of the details plus an audio file where I will talk you through the exercise to support your practice and progress.

Chapter 2: Getting Started
The Simple Version.

Standing up:

1. Pick a firm c, straight-backed chair with arm rests (figure 1).
2. Scoot forward in the chair (figure 2).
3. Place the feet straight forward and hip to shoulder width apart, ideally right under the knees (figure 2 & 3).
4. Hinge forward at the hips & roll the pelvis forward with the back flat or slightly arched (figure 4).
5. Press down with the arms to bring your weight forward and up (figure 5).
6. Engage the leg muscles (especially the glutes/buttock muscles) to lift up the rest of the way to standing (figures 6 & 7).

Sitting Down:

1. Bring the backs of the legs against the chair.
2. Hinge forward at the hips.
3. Keep the back flat or slightly arched.
4. Bend the knees and bring the buttocks back onto the seat.
5. Use the arms to slow the descent.
6. Land VERY softly on the chair-minimize "plopping".

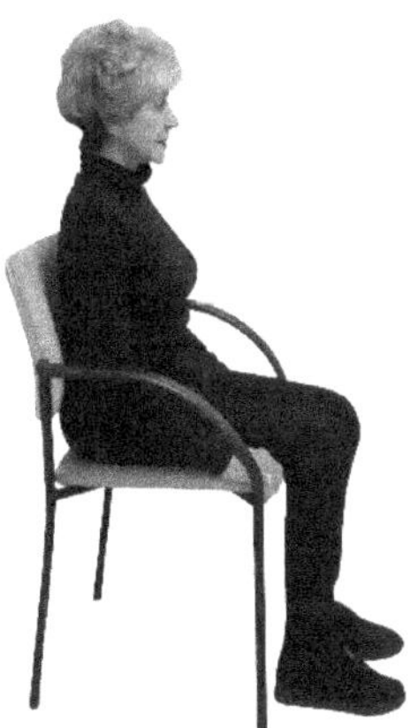

Figure 1 sitting with good posture

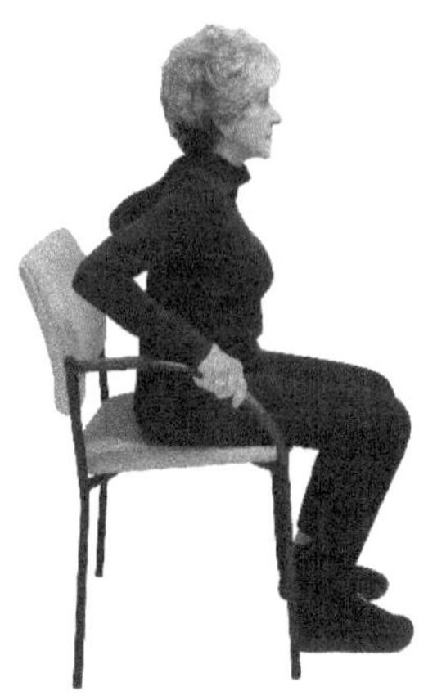

Figure 2 scooted forward in chair

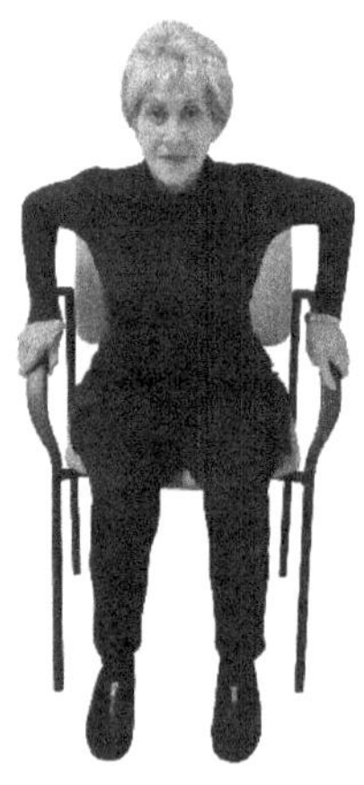

Figure 3 scooted forward in chair

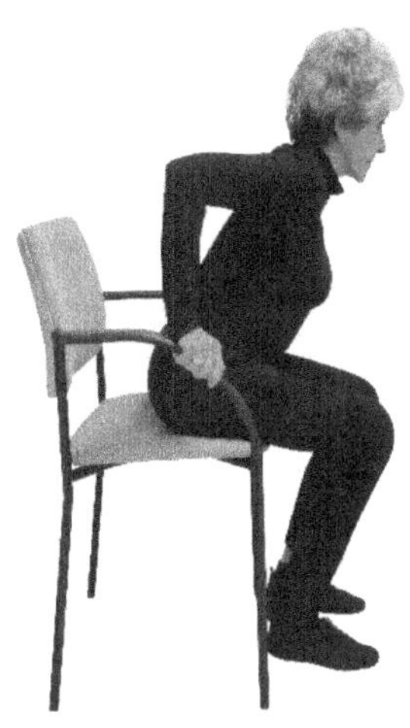

Figure 4 folding forward at hips

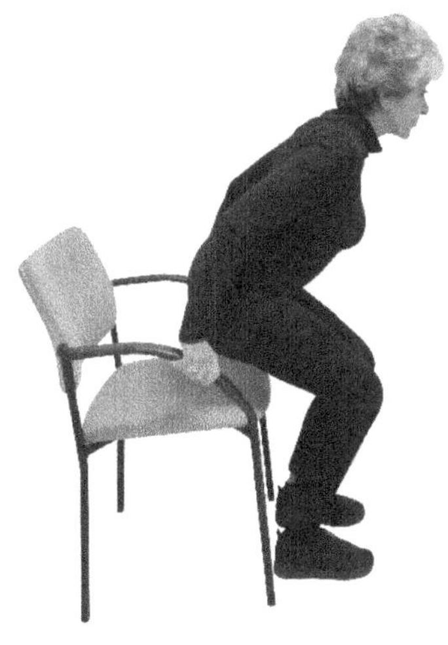

Figure 5 lift off

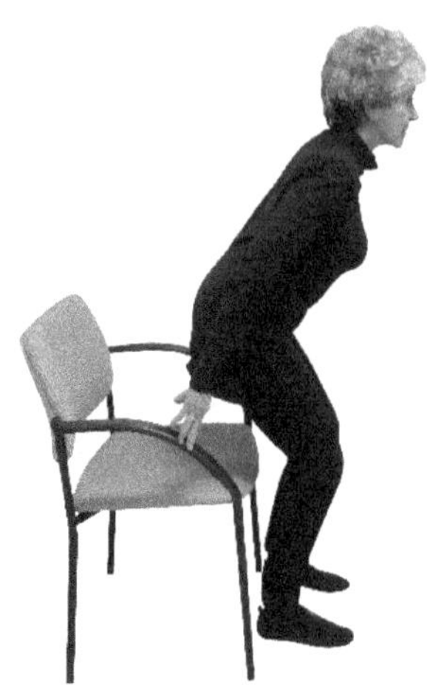

Figure 6 between lift off and standing

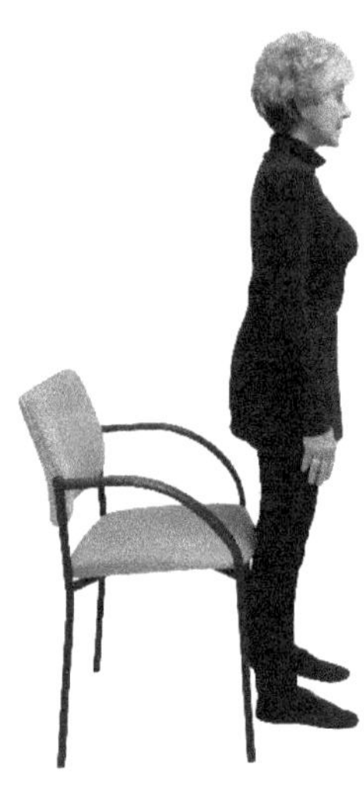

Figure 7 standing

The eyes have it

Where you look has a big impact on how easy or hard it is to get up. The direction of the gaze affects the position of the head, which, in turn, affects the whole spine. Try again with emphasis on where you are looking at each phase.

Standing up:

1. Scoot forward in the chair.
2. Place the feet straight forward and hip to shoulder width apart, ideally right under the knees.
3. Hinge forward at the hips & roll the pelvis forward with the back flat or slightly arched **(look down toward**

floor right in front of you).

4. Press down with the arms to bring your weight forward and up (look forward and down a few feet in front of you)

5. Engage the leg muscles (especially the glutes) to lift up the rest of the way to standing (**look at something eye level in front of you)**

Sitting Down:

1. Bring the backs of the legs against the chair.

2. Hinge forward at the hips

3. Keep the back flat or slightly arched **(Look Forward)**

4. Bend the knees and bring the buttocks back onto the seat. **(Look Down a few feet in front of you)**

5. Use the arms to slow the descent **(look forward)**

6. Land VERY softly on the chair-minimize "plopping".

Chapter 3: Make it Easier

If you are able to do the exercise without pain, discomfort or feeling of instability, you might skip this chapter and go to chapter 4: How Much & When?

If you are having difficulty check yourself to see if you may be making any of these common errors:

Common Errors Sit>stand:

1. Failing to bring the buttocks forward far enough in the chair (figure 8).
2. Failing to hinge forward enough at the hips to bring the weight onto the feet (figure 9).
3. Keeping the head too far back -again the weight won't go to the feet (figure 10).

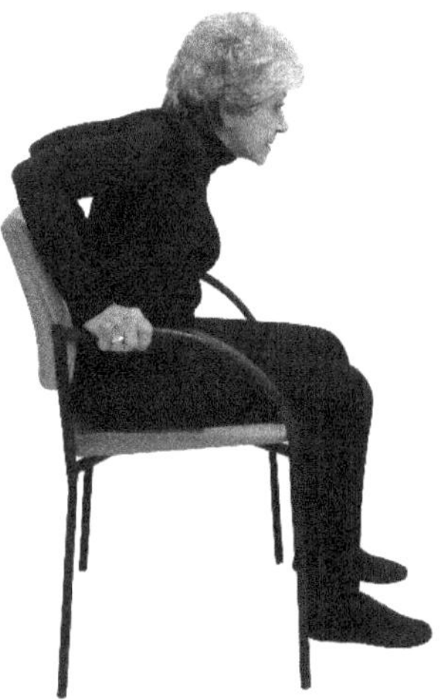

Figure 8 not scooted forward in chair

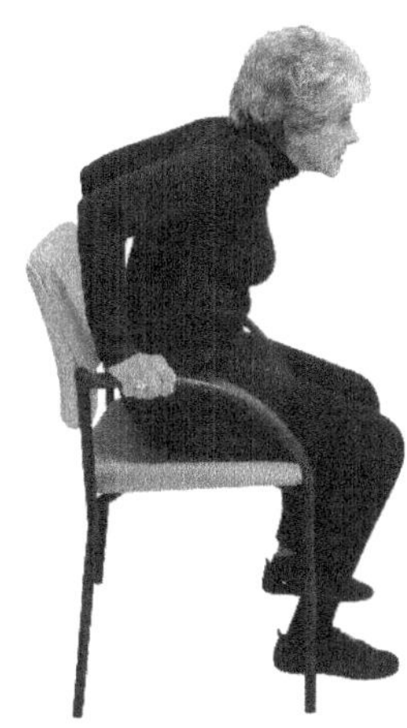

Figure 9 not hinging forward at hips

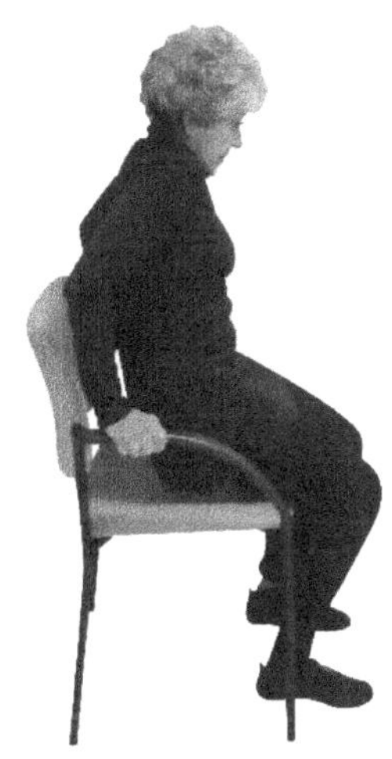

Figure 10 head too far back

Common Errors Stand > Sit

1. Not close enough to the chair -potentially catastrophic. (figure 11)

2. Not folding forward enough at the hips.

3. Over-arching or over flexing the low back. (figure 12, 13)

4. Overusing the arms to catch yourself (falling onto your hands).

5. Landing hard "Plopping".

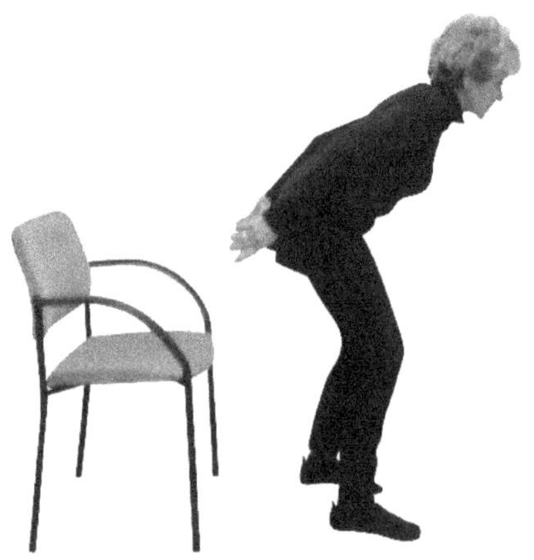

Figure 11 too far away from chair!

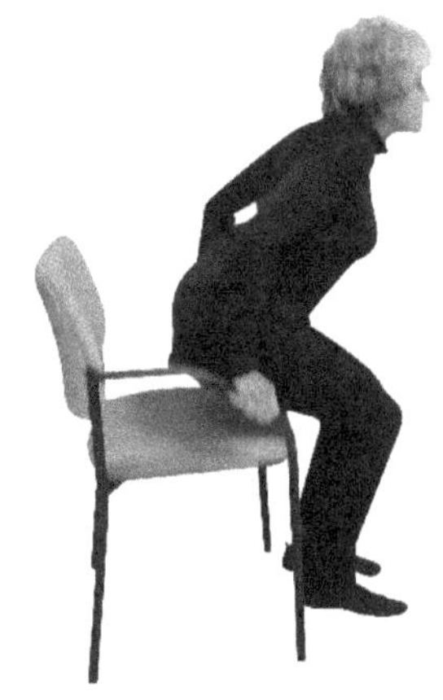

Figure 12 overarching low back

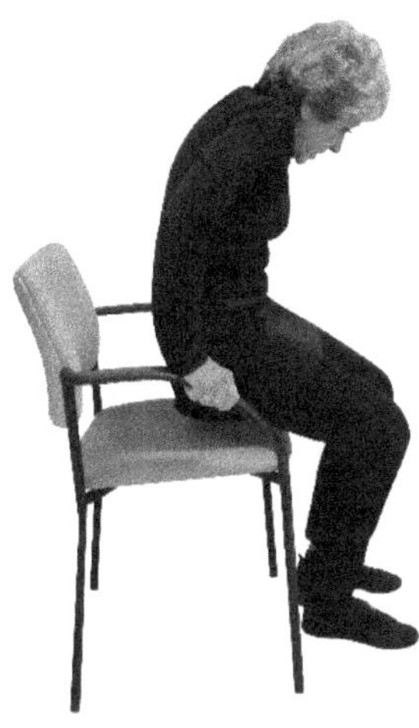

Figure 13 spine too flexed

Knee Alignment issues:

Knocked Knees

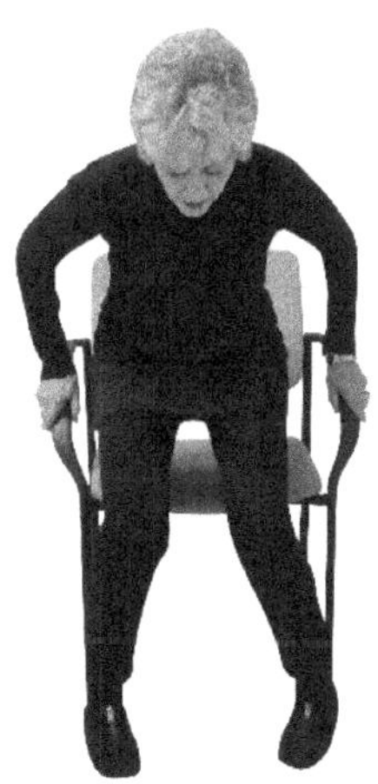

Figure 14 Knock Knees

Do your knees come close together (or even touch each other) when you go from sitting to standing? This is the most common knee alignment issue and can drive knee pain and even arthritis. It often goes with flat feet and weak gluteal muscles. Part of the reason why I recommend you point your feet straight forward (as opposed to turning them out) is that it is easier to keep the knees pointing in the same direction as the toes, if the toes are straight forward. If you find your knees rolling in while you sit↔stand, roll them out enough so that they are going in the same direction as your toes as you come up and down. Here is how to find the muscles that do this action:

1. Stand with your knees slightly flexed with toes straight forward and about shoulder width apart.
2. Imagine that you are on ice and you want to turn the toes out by pivoting on the heels-what muscles would you engage in the buttock area?
3. Since you are not on ice, the feet won't move, but the knees will roll out a bit. Find the "sweet spot" (not too much, not too little outward rotation) where the knees point in the same direction as the toes and where the knees feel most comfortable.
4. What muscles in the groin do you need to relax to allow the knees to roll out?
5. If you want to be extra-meticulous, point the knees in the direction of your second (next to the big) toe.
6. Notice that when you roll the knees out, the arches lift a bit and the inner edge of the foot gets a bit lighter on the floor, while the outer edge of the foot gets a bit heavier.

Bow Legged

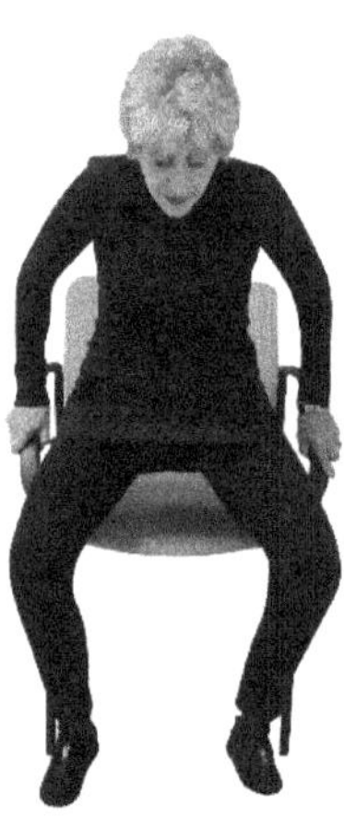

Figure 15 bow legged

Do your knees tend to roll out in relation to your toes when you are standing? This is a slightly more exotic alignment concern (compared to knock knees) and just as important to address. Here is an exploration to sort out how to fix this issue:

1. Stand with your knees slightly flexed with toes straight forward and about shoulder width apart.
2. Imagine that you are on ice and you want to turn the toes in by pivoting on the heels-what muscles would you engage in the groin area?
3. Since you are not on ice, the feet won't move, but the knees will roll in a bit. Find the "sweet spot" (not too much, not too little inward rotation) where the knees point in the same direction as the toes and where the knees feel most comfortable.
4. What muscles in buttocks do you need to relax to allow the knees to roll in?
5. If you want to be extra-meticulous, point the knees in the direction of your second (next to the big) toe.
6. Notice that when you roll the knees in, the arches drop a bit and the inner edge of the foot gets a bit heavier on

the floor, while the outer edge of the foot gets a bit lighter.

Practice to address Knock Knee & Bowlegged alignment

Whether your tendency is to roll the knees in or out, you can use the sit↔stand exercise as a way to:

1. Practice ideal knee and foot posture.
2. Strengthen muscle weakness to steer the knees correctly.
3. Lengthen and learn to relax muscles that tend to pull the knees out of alignment.

Hyperextension or Locked Knees

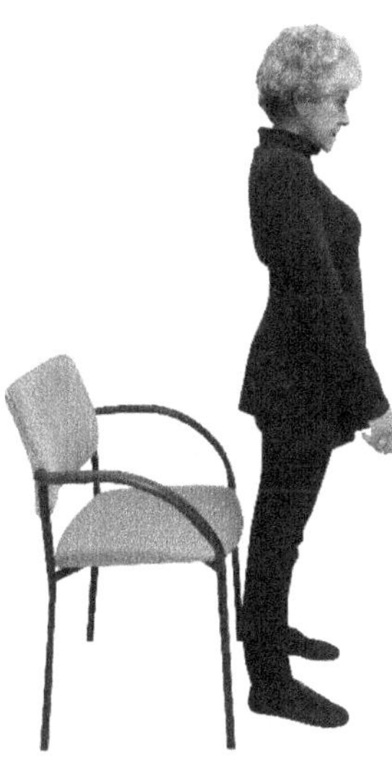

Figure 16 locked knees

Do you lock your knees to the point that they are bending backwards a bit when you stand (figure 16)? This is a very common issue that drives much of the knee, hip, pelvic and back pain that I treat on a daily basis. So far as I can tell, the only upsides to locking the knees are:

1. Energy efficiency- the leg muscles can go limp when the knees are locked.
2. Locking the knees keeps the leg from buckling when there is severe weakness.

Unless there is a famine or your legs are so weak that the only way to stand is to lock the knees, I recommend that you keep them slightly bent for the following benefits:

1. Decreased joint compression at knees.
2. Decreased joint compression at hips.
3. Decreased low back pressure.
4. Better balance from
   a. Lower center of gravity
   b. Better contact between feet and ground

5. Increased quadriceps and glute strength.
6. Better (lower & slower) breathing habits.
So, each time you come to standing, leave a hint of a bend in the knees. When you notice that your knees are locked, feel how wound up the joints feel and how less connected you are to the ground.

The Chair Matters:

We may be able to blame your difficulty with the exercise, at least in the beginning, on the chair. A straight backed, firm seated chair with solid armrests to push from is best. If you don't have a chair with arms in the home, using a solid & stable table (maybe the kitchen table) or railing (figures 17-19)to help you bring yourself up is a good option if you are having difficulty getting up without it.

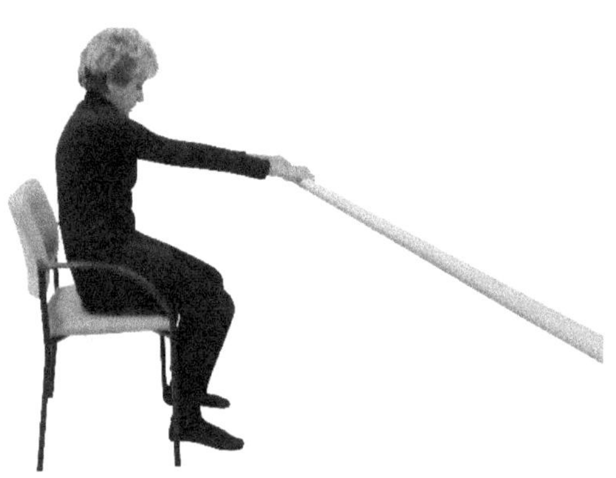

Figure 17 pulling up on railing

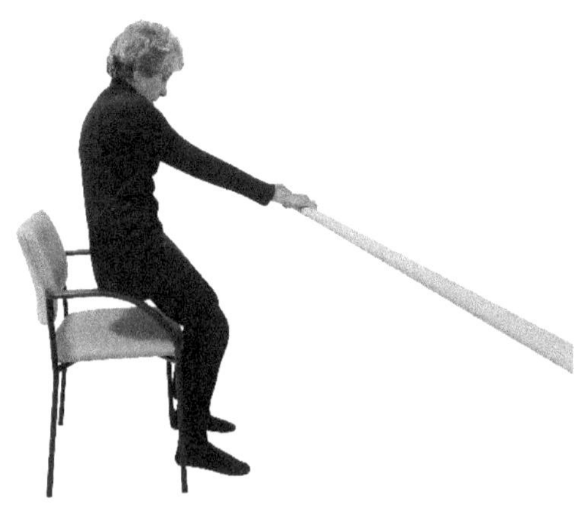

Figure 18 pulling up on railing

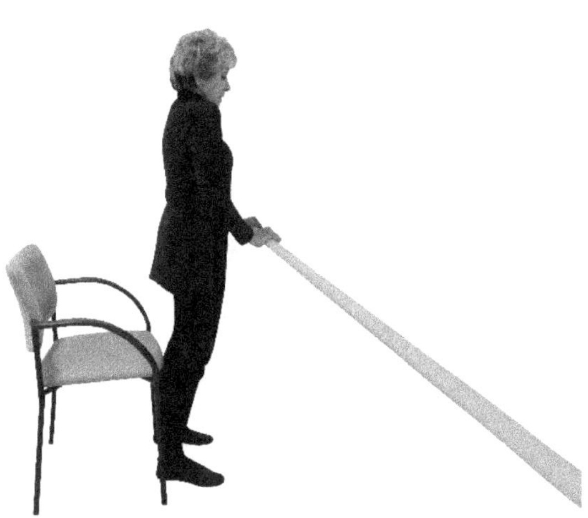

Figure 19 pulling up on railing

The higher the chair is, the easier it will be to come up and down smoothly. You may use a firm cushion or folded towel to make the seat a little higher. Sometimes a small difference in height will make a big difference in how hard it is to come up.

If the seat of the chair is tilted back (front of seat is higher than back), getting up out of it will be harder.

Another way to make it easier is to use a solid object like the edge of a sink (20, 21, 22), exposed plumbing pipe (found in city apartments-don't burn yourself if it is hot!) or bed railing to help pull yourself forward and up. This variation is particularly helpful for people who are not able to flex forward at the hips enough (say, right after a hip replacement) to bring their weight forward onto the feet enough to come up without pulling themselves forward with something. Make sure that "something" is solid! By allowing the knees to stay further back (in relation to the ankle and hips), this variation may reduce knee pain. If this is the only way to do the exercise without irritating the knees, do this version till you are able to do other variations pain free.

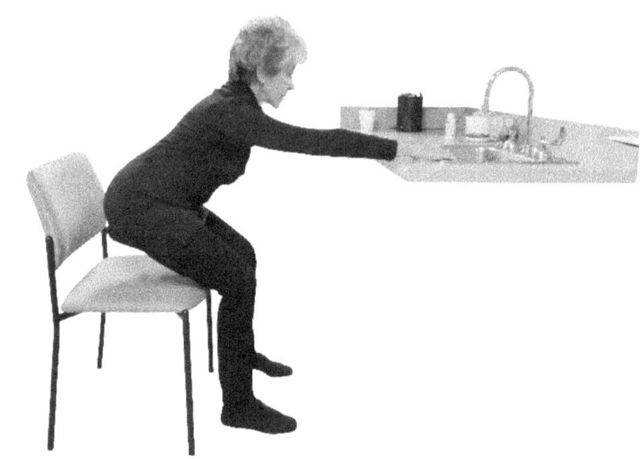

Figure 20 pulling up on sink

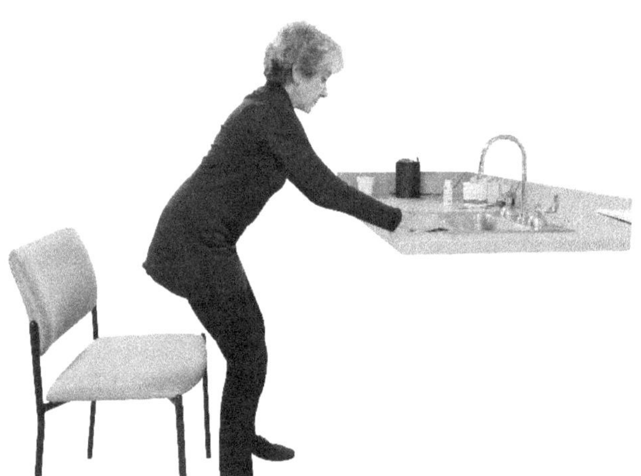

Figure 21 pulling up on sink

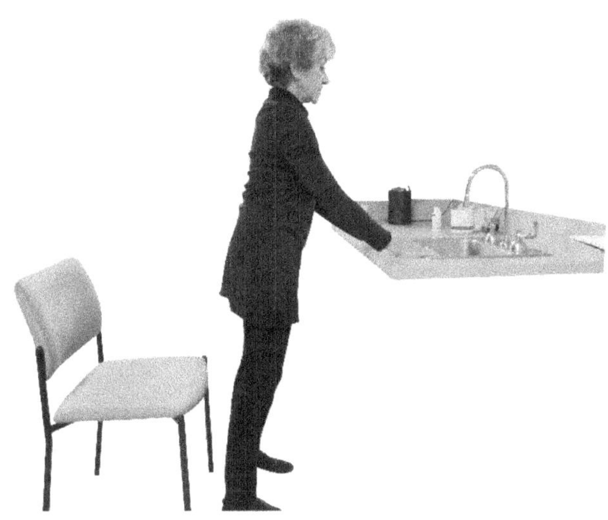

Figure 22 pulling up on sink

Foot placement:

If your feet are too far forward, it is harder to transfer the weight from your butt to your feet. Bringing the feet back till they are almost under the chair will make it easier to shift the weight of the body onto the feet so that you can use your powerful leg muscles to power the sit>stand.

Ideally, keep the toes straight forward.

Often, one leg is stronger than the other. To make it easier for today, put the weaker leg forward and put the stronger leg further back. If you have knee pain on one side, try putting that foot a bit further forward than the other to take some of the pressure off of that knee. (23)

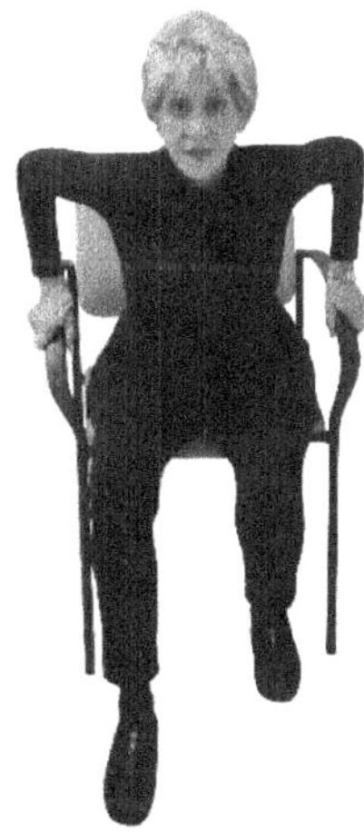

Figure 23 staggered foot position

Spinal & Pelvic Position:

If you bend forward in your low back (aka slumped position), it will be much harder to stand up (or come down smoothly) than if you keep your low back straight or very slightly arched and the pelvis rolled forward. Over-arching the back is likely to irritate the low back, especially if you have spinal stenosis, spondylolisthesis (easy for you to say:) or other conditions that make the back more sensitive to back bending. **See Chapter 6: What time is my Pelvis at?** for more on this.

19

Chapter 4: When and how many?

To benefit from the exercise you need to:

1. Do it consistently. Once in a while (or for that matter, "every now and then", "from time to time" or "occasionally") won't cut if you want the exercise to make a big difference in your life. Put it in your calendar and on your "to do" list. Tell the people who most care about you that you intend to do it regularly. Make the stakes of blowing it off high enough to keep at it because the stakes are, in fact, high. Remember how much you like to use the toilet whenever you feel the urge to......
2. Do it enough times at each session to "push the envelope" enough to get your body (brain & muscles) to adapt to the challenge.

If you do the exercise once or twice for a few times each, you will not achieve any of your goals. It needs to be done consistently and with enough repetitions each time to really tire out the key muscles that do the work. Here is a scheme that has worked for many of my clients over the years:

When? Before each meal

Building the good Habit:

By "hooking" this exercise onto a habit that most of us have (eating a few meals per day); you can do it consistently enough to make a difference in your life.

If you smoked cigarettes in the past and gave it up, you probably remember how certain activities gave you the urge to smoke again. Drinking alcohol, talking on the phone, or after a meal or sex are examples of these activities that you might have come to associate with smoking because you habitually paired the two activities.

You probably brushed your teeth this morning and you probably did it in between two other morning routine activities. You may not even remember brushing your teeth because you did it on "autopilot". You probably did not think much about it. You did not debate with yourself whether the teeth really needed it today. You just did it out of healthy habit. While I would prefer you do the exercise mindfully (more on that in **Chapter 8: What to do with the mind?**) rather than "autopilot", I would like you to cultivate a strong enough habit that you don't bother to debate with yourself whether you are going to bother with the exercise on a given day.

Physiological Reasons to Exercise Before Eating:

When the stomach is empty, there is more blood and energy available to the muscles to power the exercise, so you will be able to put more "oomph" (sorry to be so technical) into the exercise. By doing the exercise before you eat, you are likely to enhance your hormonal profile (testosterone and growth hormone) whether you are male or female for faster progress and enhanced vitality. You are also making your muscles more sensitive to the insulin that your pancreas will secrete when you eat the meal. This lets more of the nutrition end up in the muscle (especially the ones you work in the exercise) instead of enlarging fat cells.

How many? Until you are "moderately" fatigued.

I am about to give away a trade secret. Please don't tell the other physical therapists or occupational therapists that I told you this. Between you, me and the lamppost, (stage whisper) NOTHING MAGICAL HAPPENS AT TEN.

 For an exercise like sit↔stand, the main goal is to build strength and endurance. To do that, you must do enough repetitions to fatigue the muscles. When the muscles are worked enough to tire them out, you are doing microscopic damage to the muscle fibers. When you work hard enough, to cause this microtrauma, you spur the muscles on to repair the damaged fibers with bigger, stronger fibers. You also create the conditions for the nervous system (brain, spinal cord, peripheral nerves) to "learn" to do a better job of controlling those impressive muscles of yours. In other words, you need to "push the envelope" gently to enhance the hardware (muscles) and software (nervous system).

It is highly unlikely that 10 is the right number of repetitions to do for any particular exercise that is meant to build strength. It may be too many or (a better problem) too few. Rather than starting with a preconceived notion about how many is ideal, pay attention to how you feel as you continue and stop when you feel "moderately fatigued".

What the hell does "moderately fatigued" mean?

This is a moving target for a few reasons:

1. As you continue to do the exercise, your muscles will get stronger and your endurance will increase so it will take more work to fatigue them.
2. As you continue the exercise (you are going to continue aren't you?) your brain and the rest of the nervous system will get better at it.
3. As you continue to do the exercise (consistently and intensely enough) you will be able to tolerate more discomfort that comes with "pushing the envelope" allowing you to work harder. In other words, the internal yardstick for "moderately fatigued" will change in a helpful direction.

You did not really answer the Question!

I have said too much already....

Should I count or just do it till I feel it is "enough"?

I recommend that you count the repetitions each time you do the exercise and put it on a chart (Link to chart on website) and put the chart on your refrigerator door or some other place that you see it often. I particularly like the refrigerator door because it will be harder to "forget" (also known as blowing it off:) the exercise if you are reminded of it each time you get some kale, tofu or blueberries out of the fridge.

Keeping track of it has two big upsides:

1. You get to see your progress and this helps keep you motivated.
2. If you know you did 18 repetitions yesterday before breakfast and nothing terrible happened (you can still walk despite the delayed onset muscle soreness that comes 24-48 hours after you work enough to make progress), you might push yourself to hit the 20 rep mark today. Just don't rest on your laurels at 20 reps.

Isn't 20 enough? When do I get to stop progressing?

NO. More is better. NEVER.

 I have a 95 year old patient who can do 100 sit↔stand in a session with me. It helps that while he is doing the 100th rep he does not remember that it is the 100th. Remember my riff about this being about maintaining the ability to get out of a chair under your own power so that you can use the toilet anytime you like? If you are using 99% of your strength to get out of a chair or off the toilet and you lose 2% of your strength due to injury or illness, you get to experience dependence and disability. In one study done in the 50's, people on bed rest lost 1 percent of their muscle strength and mass per day so this is not an unlikely thing to happen to you. If you are using 12% of your strength to get off the toilet, you have to lose a lot more than 2% of your strength to have to wait for someone (nurse, aide or family member) to help you get to the toilet. The more repetitions you can do without stopping the more surplus strength you have to lose before you become dependent. My 95 year old client has enough surplus strength to weather a significant setback without losing his ability to move around on his own. I recommend that you keep working at improving <u>forever</u>. On the other hand, I do acknowledge a touch of bias here in my worldview. I realize that there must be a threshold of diminishing returns beyond which improvement in your ability to do the exercise without resting becomes less important. No one can really know for sure where that threshold is and I see it as more of a theoretical problem than real-world. In the real world, more is better.

Want to see how your performance measures up against other men and women in your age bracket? There are at least seven sit↔stand tests used in the scientific literature:

A. Five times stand test
B. Ten Times Stand Test
C. Single leg sit-to-stand test
D. 1-minute sit-to-stand test
E. 10 Second Sit to Stand Test
F. Six Times Sit to Stand Test
G. 30 second sit to stand
The 30 second test has normative values for people aged 60-94 and is very simple to take. You must be able to sit↔Stand without using the arms for this test to be valid for you. You just need an assistant to act as "timekeeper".

 Instructions:

1. Sit in the middle of the chair.

2. Place each hand on the opposite shoulder crossed at the wrists.

3. Place your feet flat on the floor.

4. Keep your back straight and keep your arms against your chest.

5. On "Go", rise to a full standing position and then sit back down again.

6. Repeat this for 30 seconds.

On "Go" begin timing the 30 second interval. Do not continue if you feel you may fall or faint during the test. Count the number of times you are able to come to a full standing position in 30 seconds and record it. If you over halfway to a standing position when 30 seconds have elapsed, count it as a "stand".

Here are the "below average", "average" (notice the wide span) and "above average" scores for men and women of various age brackets:

Men's Results

Age	below average	average	above average
60-64	< 14	14 to 19	> 19
65-69	< 12	12 to 18	> 18
70-74	< 12	12 to 17	> 17
75-79	< 11	11 to 17	> 17
80-84	< 10	10 to 15	> 15
85-89	< 8	8 to 14	> 14
90-94	< 7	7 to 12	> 12

Women's Results

Age	below average	average	above average
60-64	< 12	12 to 17	> 17
65-69	< 11	11 to 16	> 16
70-74	< 10	10 to 15	> 15
75-79	< 10	10 to 15	> 15
80-84	< 9	9 to 14	> 14
85-89	< 8	8 to 13	> 13
90-94	< 4	4 to 11	> 11

Rikli R, Jones C, Functional fitness normative scores for community-residing older adults, ages 60-94. J Aging Phys Activity 1999;7(2):162-81.

Remember, whether you are starting "below average", "average" or "below average", if you work at it consistently you will make progress. If you are 'above average", one injury or illness could land you in the "below average" category. Don't let a "this number is plenty" story stop your progress. More is better.

If you are not yet able to sit↔stand without using your arms, do the exercise (with the arms) consistently for a month and try again. I would bet heavily that you will be able to do it without using your arms because your strength and balance will improve.

Do I ever get to <u>not</u> do the exercise? What kind of Monster are You?

Here are reasons not to do the exercise:

1. If you have a big event (say a wedding) to go to that will be physically demanding, give yourself a break. The point of the exercise is to allow you to do things that you care about. Even though I have never met you, I really care about your ability to live your life with minimal disability. Never let the exercise prevent you from doing something out in the world that you care about. Those things connect you to the world and correlate (go along with) longevity and good function.

2. You suspect that the exercise is causing or exacerbating a "bad" pain. If you are feeling a "bad pain", consider doing it differently or taking a rest. Bad pain hallmarks are:
   A. Localized to a specific area.
   B. One side of the body (not symmetrical).
   C. Sharp in quality.
   D. In a joint (rather than muscles).
   E. Comes on suddenly (rather than gradually as you work to fatigue).
   F. Keeps you in bed (which may just be too much of a good pain for you to tolerate making it "bad" for today).
   G. The pain is getting worse day to day as you continue the program.

3. You are overtraining. There is an ideal amount of exercise for any particular person to do in a day/week/month/year. It is likely that most of the time you "undershoot" this on a regular basis if you are reading this book. It is possible to "overshoot" this ideal amount of exercise (and intensity matters). As the volume and intensity of the exercise increases past a certain threshold (which is different for everyone), the frequency should go down to allow more time for recovery. A good rule of thumb is that if you are able to do more than 100 repetitions in a day, give yourself a day of relative rest (not bed rest!) to recover before doing it again. Know that you may need to go to this one day on, one day off scheme before you get to 100 if you are dealing with any significant health issue. Another option is to have a hard day, easy day pattern where you alternate 30 rep days with 100+ Repetition days.

Ok, what if I wake up sore all over?

This is usually a sign that you pushed yourself enough to make a difference. Bravo!

Here are hallmarks of "good" pain:

1. Comes on gradually as you are exercising in muscles that are working hard.
2. Diffuse ache or soreness in the muscles you exercised recently.
3. On both sides of the body (assuming both sides of the body were worked). Symmetry is good.
4. Gets better with body warm-up and movement.
5. Over time it decreases unless you drastically increase the volume or intensity (or decrease rest).
If the pain you experience seems to meet the criteria for "bad" pain (see above), by all means, give it a rest and see a physical therapist, occupational therapist, shaman or your doctor.

Chapter 5: Making it Harder

Not hard enough for you? Here are some ideas to make you regret saying that!

The Chair:

1. Lower is harder. Work on lower surfaces till you feel comfortable getting up off the low mushy couch at the cocktail party.
2. While we are on the party theme, practice getting up with a cup of water in one hand till you feel comfortable getting up off the low surface with a glass of red wine in your hand with a white carpet on the floor.
3. A backward tilted chair (front of seat is higher than back of seat pan) will make the exercise a bit harder.
4. No armrest, or just don't use the arms. You can start the exercise not using the arms, then when you are not able to get up again without using the arms, use the arms.

Arm position (Easy to Hard)

A. Push with arms (24).
B. Reach forward with arms (25).
C. Cross arms across chest (26).

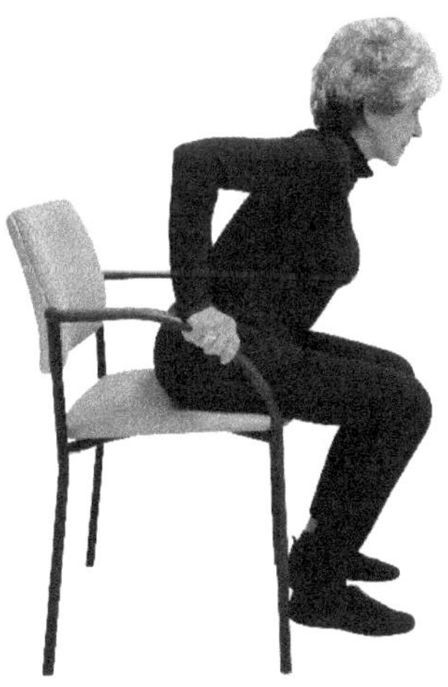

Figure 24 pushing up

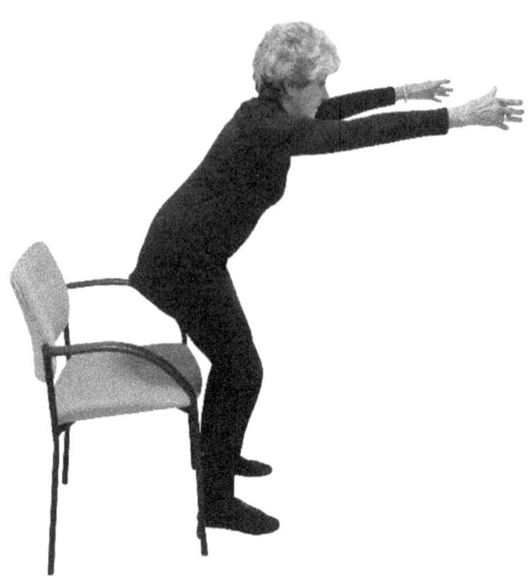

Figure 25 reaching forward

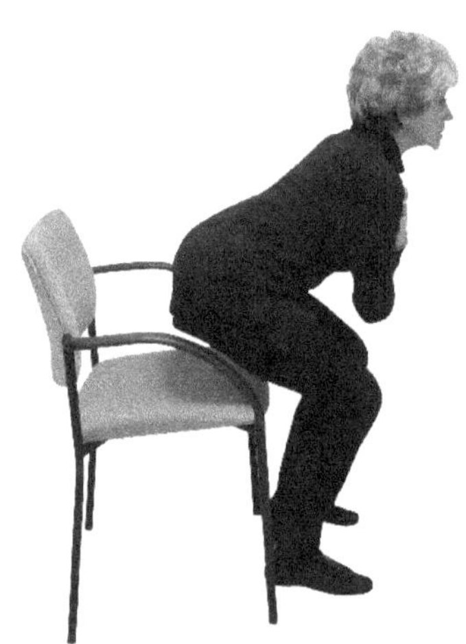

Figure 26 arms crossed

You may be able start a session with the arms crossed (hardest), then, when the legs get tired, do some repetitions of the reach forward version, then, when you need to, use the arms to help power you up.

Foot placement:

If you have been practicing (I hope!) the exercise rather than just reading this for intellectual curiosity, you have noticed that there is a "sweet spot" for the feet. Like goldilocks, you like the feet not too far forward, not too far back, not to wide, not too narrow. To make it harder and to increase your ability to deal with obstacles and conditions that dictate where you put your feet you can:

1. Put the feet farther apart than the normal "sweet spot". (figure 27)
2. Put the feet closer together. Note that this will make balance harder too as your base of support is smaller. (figure 28)

3. Put the feet further away from the chair.
4. Strong leg foot forward, weaker leg foot back (figure 29).

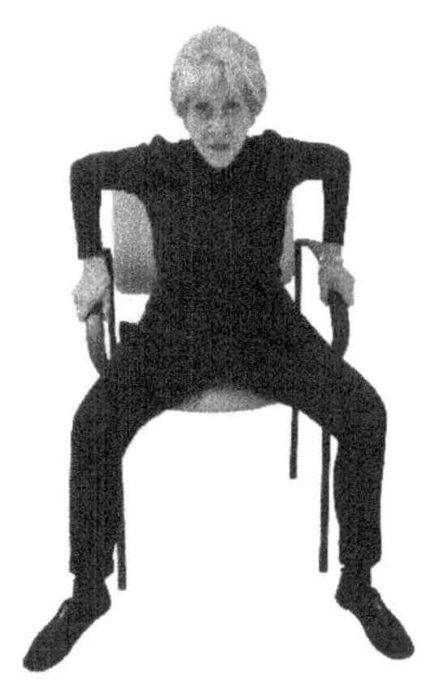

Figure 27 feet wide apart

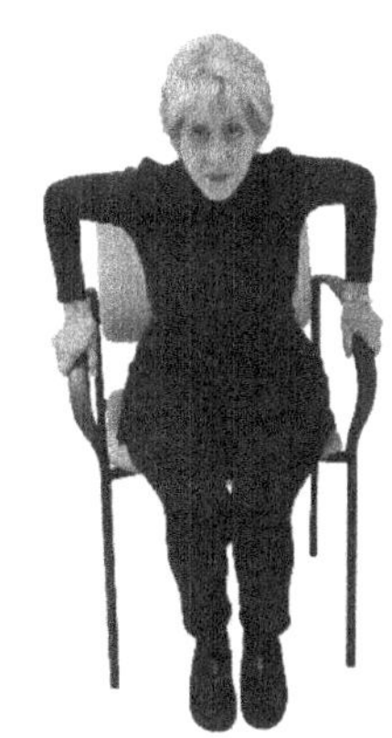

Figure 28 feet close together

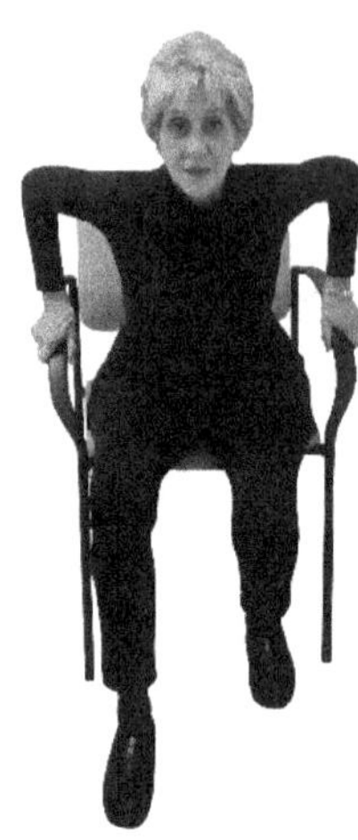

Figure 29 staggered foot placement

Often, one leg is stronger than the other. To make it harder for the weaker leg, put the stronger leg forward and put the weaker leg further back.

Other ways to make it harder:

1. Hold a weight (dumbbell [figure 30], kettlebell, water bottle, small dog or child). Notice how holding the weight more forward makes it so you don't have to flex as far forward.
2. Wear a weighted vest (I have one that I bring to particularly lucky patient's homes).
3. Slow it down a bit. There is a "preferred speed" which is probably the easiest. Slowing it down appreciably (think tai chi) makes you work much harder.
4. Speed up the sit>stand, keeping stand>sit relatively slow to build muscle power.
5. Cross your arms against your chest.
6. Close your eyes (only if your doctor and attorney agree that this is a good idea).
7. Hold a cup of water in one hand. Try not to spill any when you go up and down (figure 31).

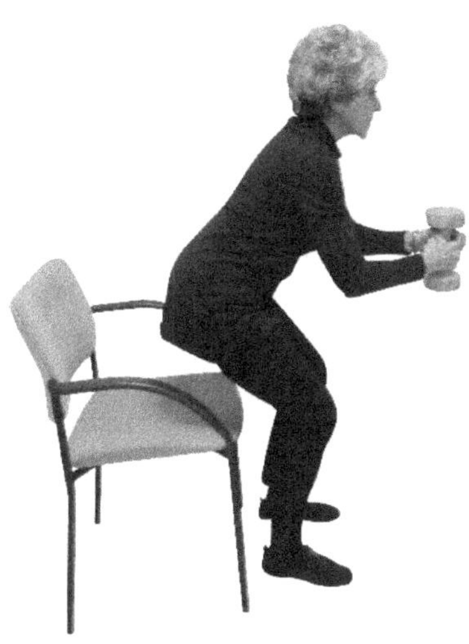

Figure 30 Holding 10 lb. weight

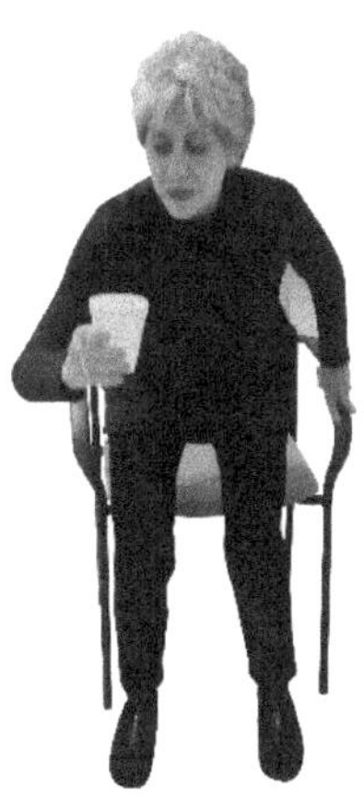

Figure 31 holding cup

Chapter 6: What Time is My Pelvis?

In my considerable experience, most people are pretty disconnected from their pelvis. This is worth addressing because besides making sit↔stand much harder or impossible, sub-optimal pelvic positioning is the root of many conditions that cause hip pain, back pain, knee pain, urological issues and sexual dysfunction. The pelvis is shaped like a bony bowl composed of three bones (IMAGE), the two innominates (left and right side) and the sacrum which fits between the innominates like a keystone. The sacrum is literally the base of the spine. "Steer" the sacrum incorrectly and the whole spine ends up in an awkward position.

The main movement of the pelvis that I would like to focus on here for the purpose of this particular exercise, is forward rotation (front goes down, back goes up) and backward rotation (front goes up, back goes down).

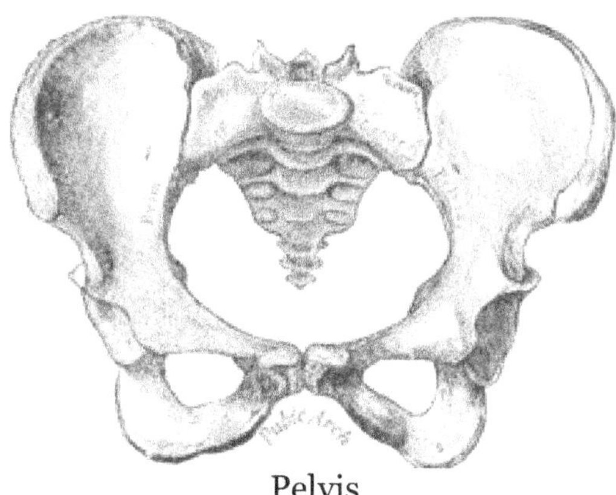

Pelvis

Go ahead and find your navel. Palpate yourself down below the navel till you find the Pubic Arch, where the two sides of the pelvis come together with a rubbery cartilage joint. Then palpate out along the bone till you feel the iliac crest, which goes higher as you feel it from front to back. If you can comfortably reach the back of the pelvis, feel where the tailbone ends. Then, unless your hands are fragile, sit on them to feel the rounded protuberance (SITS bone) that (ideally) we balance our weight on when we sit. Gently rock the pelvis forward and back to feel how it moves the weight in the direction that you roll it in.

Imagine that the pelvis is a bowl and you are sitting on a clock. The clock is oriented with 12:00 forward and 6:00 backward. When you are rolling the pelvis forward on the hip joint, you are bringing it toward 12:00. This 6/12 language comes from Moshe Feldenkrais, who devised a brilliant way to bring awareness to pelvic movement options.

Keeping the movement small enough and slow enough to be totally comfortable and easy, roll the pelvis forward

(12:00-figure 32) and back (6:00-figure 34). Notice how the movement ripples up the spine arching the back at 12:00 and bending forward at 6:00. Feel how the chin gets farther from the chest at 12:00 and closer to the chest at 6:00.

It is "mission critical" that the pelvis roll forward sufficiently to achieve sit↔stand elegantly. Yes, "elegance" is a potential bonus upside from reading (and practicing the exercise in) this book!

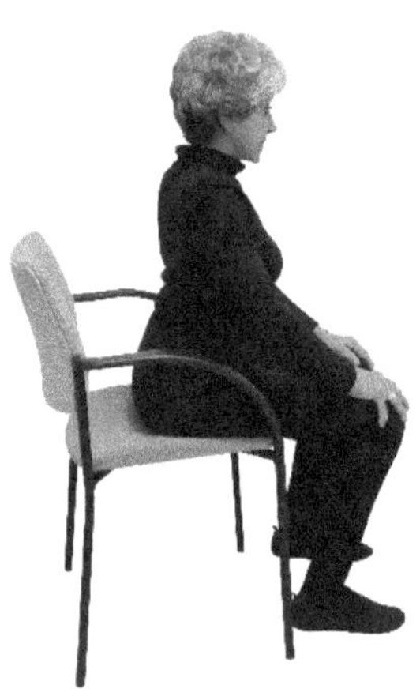

Figure 32 12:00

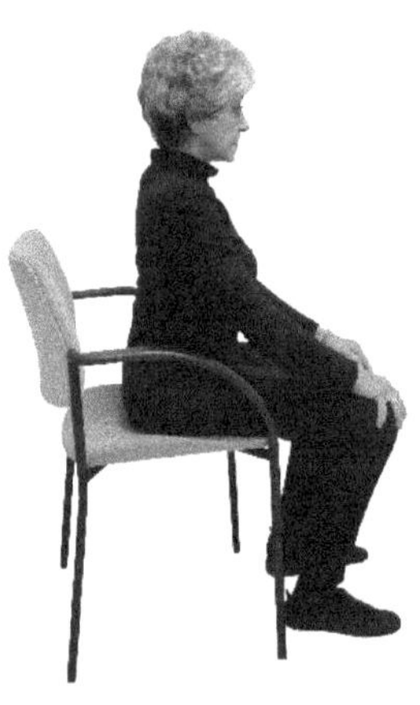

Figure 33 Neutral

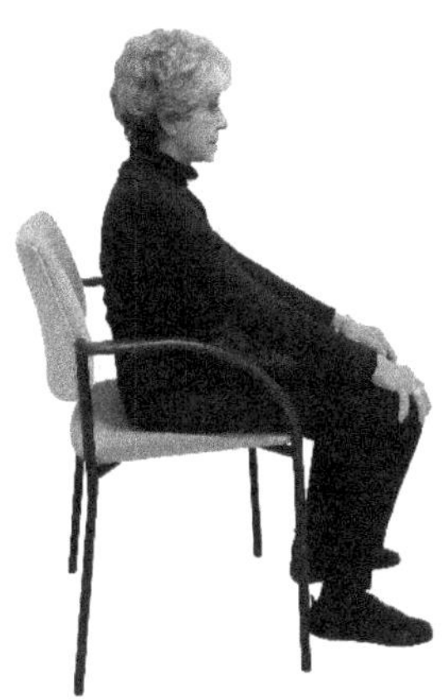

Figure 34 6:00

Hamstrings and pelvic tilt forward toward 12:00

If you are having trouble folding forward at the hips and rolling the pelvis toward 12:00 (and feel tightness behind the knee(s), your hamstrings may be too tight for optimal function. You can do a hamstring stretch right from that chair (figure 35) you are having trouble getting out of because of them. Straighten one leg in front of you, reaching the heel as far away as possible. Keep the other knee bent about 90 degrees, sit tall and hinge forward at the hips till you feel a strong but not painful pulling sensation behind the knees. Hang out in the stretch zone for about a minute, and then switch sides. If one side is way tighter, consider giving that one a double dose.

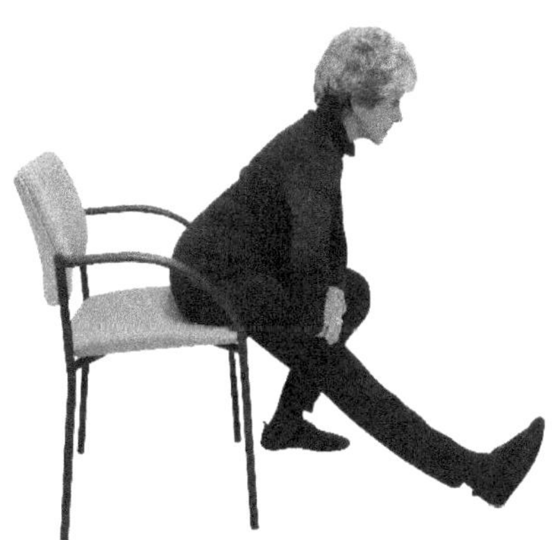

Figure 35 hamstring stretch

After all of this pelvic exploration and tinkering, let's try a few repetitions to see if you notice a difference when you focus on the pelvis more.

Standing up:

1. Pick a firm cushioned, straight-backed chair with arm rests.
2. Scoot forward in the chair.
3. Place the feet straight forward hip to shoulder width apart
4. Sit Tall **(pelvis and low back in neutral position)**
5. Hinge forward at the hips & **roll the pelvis** forward with the back flat or slightly arched (look down toward floor right in front of you).
6. Press down with the arms to bring your weight forward and up (look forward and down a few feet in front of you)
7. Engage the leg muscles (especially the glutes) to lift up the rest of the way to standing, while **rolling the pelvis back slightly** (look at something eye level in front of you)
Sitting Down:

1. Bring the backs of the legs against the chair.
2. Hinge forward at the hips **(roll the pelvis forward)**
3. Keep the back flat or slightly arched
4. Bend the knees and bring the buttocks back onto the seat.
5. Use the arms to slow the descent
6. Land VERY softly on the chair-minimize "plopping".
7. Roll the pelvis back to sit tall and relaxed.

What if 6:00 or 12:00 hurts?

I like to tell my patients "if you see the hornet's nest, don't poke at it". If 6:00 or (more likely) 12:00 is painful, don't keep going into the painful direction. Pay attention to how far you can go in that direction (which may be not at all) before the discomfort starts.

Often, by moving the pelvis in the pain-free range of motion, a painful part of the pelvic clock becomes pain free. This improvement is caused by some combination of mechanical effects (e.g. joint mobilization) and neural adaptation (learning).

If you find that this action of gently rolling the pelvis forward and back loosens the hips, pelvis and spine in a way that decreases pain or stiffness, consider doing it before rising whenever you have been sitting for a long time.

1. Check at the restaurant is coming-Do the pelvic clock.
2. Credits are rolling after the movie-Do the pelvic clock.
3. The plane is descending-Do the pelvic clock.

Chapter 7: What to do with The Breath?

Every "breathing" muscle is also involved with sit↔stand. Most people who I work with are not breathing efficiently and that can cause premature fatigue or even the inability to get out of a chair on their own. By coordinating your breath with the sequence of movements to sit↔stand, you can increase your capacity and make it more comfortable and easy to accomplish. Whenever you work with the breath, I recommend being gentle and have an experimental and explorative mindset. Rather than working hard to "get it right", play with the ideas below and look for ease in the breath and the exercise.

Breathing Pattern #1

Standing up:

1. Sit tall and Exhale.
2. Inhale while you Hinge forward at the hips with the back flat or slightly arched.
3. Exhale as you Press down with the arms to bring your weight forward and up.
4. Inhale as you Engage the leg muscles (especially the glutes) to lift up the rest of the way to standing.

Sitting Down:

1. Make sure the backs of the legs are against the chair.
2. *Inhale* as you Hinge forward at the hips & Keep the back flat or slightly arched.
3. *Exhale* as you Bend the knees and bring the buttocks back onto the seat.
4. Use the arms to slow the descent.
5. Land VERY softly on the chair-minimize "plopping".
6. *Inhale* as you settle into the chair.

Rather than "locking" the breath to the movement in the above pattern as if it were the "tablet brought down from the mountain", use is as a good place to start the experimental exploration of how to let your breathing pattern be in harmony with the sit↔stand exercise.

You may very well find that, depending on the situation, different patterns of coordination between the movement and breath serve you better.

Here is another pattern to play with:

Breathing Pattern #2:

1. Sit tall and *Inhale.*
2. Fold forward and *Exhale.*
3. Lift off>stand *Inhale.*
4. Fold Forward *Exhale.*

5. Sit tall and Inhale
And another:

Breathing pattern #3:

1. Sit tall _Exhale._
2. Fold forward _Inhale._
3. Lift off to stand _Exhale._
4. Fold (to sit) forward _Inhale._
5. Sit tall (exhale)-back to # 2 (fold forward and inhale)
 Which pattern feels easiest? Which feels hardest? Spend most of your time practicing the pattern that feels most congruent with the exercise and makes it relatively easy and comfortable.

Chapter 8: What to do with the Mind?

If you listen to the radio or make "to do" lists while you do the exercise, you will benefit from the exercise. If you pay attention to the sensations elicited by sit↔stand, you will also get the following benefits:

1. You are less likely to do something "wrong" that causes pain ("bad pain" see chapter 4) during the exercise.
2. You are more likely to learn from the work how to optimize your performance.
3. Improved balance
4. You get the benefits of meditation:
 A. Decreased anxiety
 B. Improved immune function.
 C. Better digestion.
 D. Improved cognition.
 E. Enhanced ability to empathize and improve relationships with people in your life.
 F. Better brain circuitry for controlling the body.
Better what?

There is plenty of evidence that when we pay attention to the body as we move it, we are laying down new nerve cells in the brain and elsewhere that enhance brain power.

So what exactly am I suggesting?

1. While doing the sit↔stand exercise (or any other exercise for that matter) pay attention to the sensations you experience.
2. Rather than judging the sensations as "good" or "bad" (within reason-see hallmarks of bad pains that should get you to stop what you are doing), simply feel what you feel.
 a. Sensations of movement and pressure change with the breath.
 b. Sensations of movement and pressure change as you move the body.
 c. Sensations of the muscles working to sit↔stand.
 d. What you see (with the eyes) as you do the workout.
 e. What you hear as you do the workout.
3. When (not if) the mind wanders, bring it back to sensations in the present moment.
4. Notice how you feel before the exercise and how you feel after you have done a round of it. What is the difference? Physical changes? Mental clarity changes? Mood changes?
It is ok to spend some time experimenting and analyzing your movement pattern details, but spend most of the time simply resting the mind in the activity. Many people who exercise regularly do it not because of all the things that they know it is good for them. They do it because they crave the sensations and feelings that the

exercise elicits and promotes. If you never pay enough attention to notice these effects, you are less likely to cultivate a habit of doing the exercise.

Pay attention to the sensations to help yourself get "hooked" on exercise.

Chapter 9: Motivation & Next Steps

Motivation

People who have trouble with sit↔stand are more likely to fall while coming up (especially when absent minded) or while walking. They are more likely to need help with basic daily tasks (dressing, toileting, meal preparation). They are also more likely to die in the not-too-distant-future. For the vast majority of people, there is nothing "in the way" of going in another direction. Nothing in the way except self-limiting beliefs that are potentially, self-fulfilling prophesies.

Rather than buying into all these self-limiting "stories" that you tell yourself, give letting one go a try. Let go of the "I am not an exerciser" story. Let that story die so that you can live a longer, more independent, more comfortable life.

Write yourself (or tell someone) a new "Story". Imagine that you read this book a year ago and that you followed all the recommendations in it. Write or tell the story as if you were praising yourself and the exercise's ability to improve items below that you are hoping to address:

1. Your ability to stand up from a variety of chairs.
2. Your strength and endurance in general.
3. Your willpower/ability to stick with an exercise long enough to benefit from it.
4. Your mood.
5. Your body composition (less fat, more muscle, denser bone).
6. Your ability to deal with physical and mental stress.
7. Your sleep quality which in turn improves mood, cognition, eating habits, immune function.
8. Your cognition.
9. Your sexual function.

Write or tell the story as if these improvements had already happened. Along with writing or telling the story, imagine how you will feel in your body and mind after doing the exercise consistently for one year.

Tactics to Stay Motivated:

1. Put it in your calendar and on your "to do" lists.
2. Tell the people who most care about you that you intend to do it regularly. Be specific.
3. Keep track of your performance and prominently display the chart.

Next Steps

Is sit↔stand the only exercise worth doing?

The best exercise is the one (or more) that you *actually do* and the biggest problem with exercise is that you don't do it. This book focuses on one particular exercise that is super-functional and works the whole body. There are many other useful exercises including walking, Tai Chi, Yoga and weight-lifting. Part of the idea behind this book is that people are less likely to do exercise if they see it as overwhelming. When I give a patient one exercise, they are way more likely to do it than if I give them ten exercises. This program is designed to maximize your participation by making it very simple and easy to follow. I hope that after engaging in this exercise for long enough to feel the benefits, you are inspired to add other exercises to your program.

Chapter 10: Conclusion

I have approached the teaching of this simple exercise as if placing one layer after another to gradually clarify the surprising number of details to manipulate or experiment with to enhance the effects of it. Layer one was the bare bones instructions. Layer two added how to manage the gaze to promote better performance. Knee alignment formed another layer to make the exercise better for your joints and more comfortable. Next, the movement of the pelvis was explored to make sure that the body segments are oriented in the best way to easefully do the movement. The breath overlay (with multiple options) formed the fourth "layer". Layer five dealt with the mind and how to turn the exercise into a moving meditation to garner all the benefits of mindfulness. Finally, none of the previous "layers" matter if you don't actually do the exercise, so I have given you concrete ways to get and stay engaged in the exercise. You have a gauge that you can use at any time to see how your performance compares to other people of your age and gender. I have shared ways to make the act of standing up from a chair easier. I have also shown you how to keep challenging yourself with variations of the exercise for years to come.

If you have found the book helpful, please review it!

About the Author

Bill Gallagher PT, CMT, CYT

-Director of the East West Rehabilitation Institute

-Master Clinician in Integrative Rehabilitation, Mount Sinai Medical Center

-Instructor in Clinical Physical Therapy, Columbia University

-Certified Yoga Teacher

-Certified Baguazhang Teacher

-Experienced Tai Chi Teacher

-Licensed Physical Therapist

Bill Gallagher has developed a uniquely integrative approach to maximize function and prevent falls. By integrating the Physical Therapy traditions of the East (Tai Chi, Baguazhang, Qigong/Neigong, Yoga) with somatic therapies of the West (Conventional Therapeutic Exercise, Feldenkrais, Alexander, Osteopathy), Mr. Gallagher helps his clients maximize function and minimize pain.

Through meditation instruction, guided imagery and other disciplines that work with the Mind & Body, clients are further empowered to optimize function and comfort while reducing suffering.

Bill sees a broad spectrum of clients in his practice including people with severe disabilities and elite performers. In addition to typical 1:1 sessions, Bill teaches specialized group programs for people with breathing issues, spinal cord injury, brain injury, chronic pain (back pain, pelvic pain, arthritis), breast cancer survivors, and elders at risk of falling.

His work has been published in Topics in Geriatric Rehabilitation, Occupational Therapy Practice, Advance for Physical Therapists, Advance for Occupational Therapists and Tai Chi magazine.

He has also written a chapter for a physical therapy text, Complementary Therapies for Physical Therapy: A Clinical Decision-making Approach on integrating Tai Chi & Qigong with conventional physical therapy for psychological, cardiac and arthritic conditions.

Bill is recognized as an authority on Integrative/Mind-Body/Complementary rehabilitation and teaches his visionary synthesis to practicing rehab clinicians, at retreat centers and at several Physical Therapy doctoral programs including Columbia University. He has also presented at professional conferences including the World Physical Therapy Confederation, The American Physical Therapy Association, The National Association of Certified Professional Midwives, The American Occupational Therapist Association and the **Pennsylvania Association of Naturopathic**

Physicians.

Bill lives and practices in New York City

If you have found the book helpful, please review it!